T0144717

RELORA

The Natural Breakthrough to Losing Stress-Related Fat and Wrinkles

JAMES B. LAVALLE,
R.Ph., C.N.C.
With Ernest Hawkins, R.Ph.

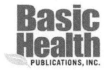

Basic
Health
PUBLICATIONS, INC.

The information contained in this book is based upon the research and personal and professional experiences of the author. It is not intended as a substitute for consulting with your physician or other healthcare provider. Any attempt to diagnose and treat an illness should be done under the direction of a healthcare professional.

The publisher does not advocate the use of any particular healthcare protocol but believes the information in this book should be available to the public. The publisher and author are not responsible for any adverse effects or consequences resulting from the use of the suggestions, preparations, or procedures discussed in this book. Should the reader have any questions concerning the appropriateness of any procedures or preparation mentioned, the author and the publisher strongly suggest consulting a professional healthcare advisor.

Series Cover Designer: Mike Stromberg
Editor: Rowan Jacobson
Typesetter: Gary A. Rosenberg

Basic Health Guides are published by
Basic Health Publications, Inc.

Contents

Introduction

We are a stressed-out society. If you are like most of us, this will come as no surprise. Stress is something all people experience at times in their lives, but in the fast-paced, technological, demanding lifestyle of the West, it has become epidemic. And whether it is due to a death in the family, relationship problems, health crises, or just simply trying to keep up with day-to-day tasks, we feel the impact of stress. You are driving down the road, late for work, and that person in front of you just won't move—stress! Your boss calls you into the office and says you need to work harder—stress! The bill collectors are calling and you don't have the money to pay them—stress! Your kids are yelling, the dog's barking, and the phone's ringing—stress! The examples are endless, but what matters is the effect all this stress has upon us.

Over the past few years, researchers have reported that feeling stressed out isn't just something in our heads, it also shows up in our bodies—and it can have deadly consequences. Recent studies have attributed over 85 percent of all diseases to stress-related factors.[1] Stress often manifests in individuals as anxiety or depression.[2] Stress causes an increase in the hormone cortisol, which causes hunger cravings and weight gain, inflammation in the joints, changes in blood sugar regulation, thyroid changes, blood pressure changes, immune system dysfunction, and other problems that will be discussed later in this booklet. Stress also decreases the hormone DHEA (dehydroepiandrosterone), which in addition to regulating sex hormones seems to slow many of the effects of aging. Clearly, our well-being depends on us getting our stress under control.

Just as stress is nothing new, neither are human beings' attempts to manage it. The Ancient Egyptians had aromatherapy oils, the Romans tried baths and lounging, the Chinese favored herbal mixtures and meditation. Modern physicians have tried to manage stress for decades with high-powered pharmaceuticals, such as Valium and Xanax, and although these drugs will cause relaxation, they often make people lethargic and unable to function normally—mentally, physically, and even sexually. They also tend to be habit-forming.

Wouldn't it be nice to find a solution to decrease that unwanted stress, along with the food cravings and weight gains it causes, and to improve your immune system and slow down the aging process as well—all without causing stupor or addiction? More and more evidence is pointing to the discovery of just such a product. It is called Relora, and it is brand new on the market.

A dietary supplement developed over a four-year period, Relora is the result of a worldwide effort to screen more than one hundred traditional medicinal ingredients for the best possible natural product for stress and cortisol control. Some of the active compounds in Relora have been studied extensively for twenty-five years, and the plants from which it is derived have been used for centuries by many cultures to support the body and nurture well-being. Relora tackles the effects of stress head-on, enhancing mental, emotional, and physical vitality, and normalizing cortisol and DHEA levels. It can even help you shed those unwanted pounds!

What Is Relora?

Relora is a proprietary product developed by Next Pharmaceuticals, Inc., a California-based research and development company specializing in natural ingredients for dietary supplements. It contains ingredients extracted from two plant species that have been used in traditional Chinese medicine for more than 1,500 years: *Phellodendron amurense* and *Magnolia officinalis*. Relora helps to relieve stress and anxiety, which in turn may help you lose weight. The research and development of Relora involved sophisticated testing and screening for ingredients that have antianxiety properties but no sedative effects.[3] Initially, investigators tested the Magnoliaceae plant family as a lead source of potential antianxiety products. Later studies on *Phellodendron amurense* led to the discovery of an extract that complements the pharmacological activity of the magnolia extract. The final formulation of Relora is a proprietary blend of the two extracts. Through a series of studies, it became clear to the scientists that Relora was a safe and effective formulation. Unlike pharmaceuticals, Relora works with the body's natural chemistry to maintain normal levels of cortisol and DHEA, hormones that, as we've seen, not only affect physical and emotional well-being but can also have a major impact on appetite and how the body metabolizes fat. By working to re-establish a stable balance of these hormones, Relora can help you break the stress cycle and restore optimum health to mind and body.

In addition to controlling mild anxiety and the symptoms associated with it—such as irritability, restlessness, tense muscles, poor sleep, fatigue, and difficulty concentrating[4]—Relora has another important benefit: it is nonsedating. The plant extracts in Relora bind directly to several important targets in the central nervous system associated with anxiety, bypassing the mechanisms involved in alertness entirely.[5]

In this booklet, we will examine what stress is—why it exists, what can trigger it, and what the deleterious effects of it are—and then go on to learn how Relora combats this killer. We will then go on to explore a complete regimen of Relora use, combined with other supplements and lifestyle changes, that can significantly reduce stress, improve appearance, and bring you many extra years of healthy living. Read on—relief is at your fingertips.

1. What Is Stress?

Stress involves anything that disturbs an individual's physical, mental, or emotional equilibrium. It can be defined as a number of normal reactions by the body (mental, emotional, and physical) that are designed for self-preservation. As such, stress is a normal, desirable, and beneficial part of our lives. Most people are more active, more invigorated, more creative, more productive, and more alive because of the challenges created by minor stresses. However, many people are also exposed to much higher levels of stress than they realize. And when the stress response is set off too often, and at improper times, it can have a detrimental effect on the body.

When the body is under stress, the nervous system responds by increasing a biochemical activity termed "sympathetic activity," which releases certain brain chemicals that create nervous restlessness, hyperactivity, anxiety, muscle tension, cardiovascular stress, and intestinal cramping, to name a few symptoms. The body has numerous stress response mechanisms and stress can affect the body in different ways. In fact, the same form of stress might cause one individual to get a migraine, a second to have an ulcer attack, and a third to have elevated blood pressure. What really matters is how much stress, what kind of stress, and, ultimately, how each individual handles his or her stresses.

During the course of hundreds of thousands of years of evolution, humans have developed an internal biochemical mechanism for dealing with stress that is referred to as the "fight or flight" response. Stressful life events—whether major, such as the loss of a loved one or a job, or routine, such as traffic jams and family disagreements—set off the release of hormones that help your body charge up to meet the challenge. Your pupils widen to let in more light. Your alertness increases because of more neurochemicals released in your brain. Your adrenal glands begin to pump epinephrine and cortisol into your bloodstream. Your heart races, your blood pressure rises, your muscles tense. Your liver starts converting starches to sugars for energy, and digestion slows. Experts have even determined that your blood's clotting powers are enhanced during stressful situations, just in case of blood loss. Sweat production increases and the hair on your body may feel prickly and actually stand on end. Obviously, these physiological changes can be very useful if the body needs to use extra resources to quickly resolve an important situation. But when these same protective hormones are produced repeatedly, or in excess, because of constant stressful events, they create a gradual and steady cascade of harmful physiological changes, wearing the body out.

An example of the initial, or *alarm stage* of stress may occur after intense exercise that causes a stiffness or soreness to develop in overworked muscles. Under normal conditions, these symptoms will subside and the muscle will return to its normal state within a day or two. However, if the muscle continues to be overworked, or is exposed to additional stresses, the body engages in the *resistance stage*. At this point, the body tries to adapt to the repetitive stress factors that are making excess demands on it. This stage of adaptation may last for years as the body tries to find ways to cope with the unusual levels of chronic stress. It might involve changes in the liver, pancreas, or cardiovascular system. Weight gain may also occur. Numerous biochemical and nutritional factors may come into play. Or, in the case of the above-mentioned stressed muscle, the changes might involve the tendons, ligaments, and skeletal alignment.

When our bodies go into the resistance stage, our health is in jeopardy. Unless we learn how to handle stress, we may become subject to its debilitating and lifelong effects. This chapter will discuss some of the physiological changes that occur when we are chronically "stressed out." By understanding them, we will be able to see why Relora can be a lifesaver for so many people. Now let's look an in-depth look at the causes of chronic stress.

WARNING SIGNS OF STRESS

- Nervousness and anxiety
- Depression
- Irritability
- Forgetfulness
- Learning difficulties
- Insomnia
- Frequent accidents
- Back pain
- Muscle tension
- Headaches
- Shaking hands
- Diarrhea
- Constipation

- Heart palpitations
- Chest pain
- Sweaty, cold hands
- Shortness of breath
- Indigestion
- Dizziness
- Frequent colds
- Ringing in the ears
- Teeth grinding
- Hives or rashes
- Loss of appetite
- Nausea or vomiting
- Stomach pain

What Causes Stress?

Many different factors can cause stress, from physical (such as an injury) to emotional and mental (fear of something dangerous, or worry over losing your job). Identifying what may be causing you stress is often the first step to learning how to better deal with it. Some of the most common sources of stress are:

Survival Stress. This is the "fight or flight" response, common in people and animals. When faced with a physical threat, your body naturally responds with a burst of energy so that you will be better able to fend off the danger (fight) or escape it altogether (flight). Hormones are what allow your body to use energy at a rate beyond its normal resting state.

Internal Stress. Have you ever caught yourself worrying about things you can do nothing about, or worrying for no reason at all? Internal stresses are some of the most important kinds of stress to understand and manage. Internal stress is when people make themselves stressed by worrying about things they can't control or putting themselves in situations they know will cause them stress. Some people become addicted to the kind of hurried, tense lifestyle that results from being under stress. They even look for stressful situations and feel stress about things that aren't stressful!

Environmental Stress. This is a physical reaction to things such as noise, drinking, crowds, climate changes, and even pressure from work or family. Excessive drug use, whether prescription, recreational, caffeine, or over-the-counter, can also stress the body. The stress of living in poverty or in an unhealthy, polluted environment has an enormous impact on health status that researchers are only just beginning to understand. A frustrating job is another leading cause of environmental stress. Identifying these environmental stresses and learning to avoid them or deal with them can help save your life.

Fatigue and Overwork. This kind of stress builds up over a long time and can take a hard toll on your body. It can be caused by working too much or too hard at your job, school, or home. It can also be caused by not knowing how to manage your time well or how to take time out for rest and relaxation. This can be one of the hardest kinds of stress to avoid because many people feel this is out of their control. Many of the stresses we have in our home life originate from our stresses generated at the workplace.

Chronic Stress

Chronic stress arises when you keep yourself in an alert state for too many hours each day. A daily regimen of racing heartbeat, pulsing blood, tensed muscles, undigested food stuck in your stomach, and elevated levels of hormones coursing through your circulatory system poses all kinds of potential health problems. Take the hormone cortisol, for instance. Cortisol is a necessary part of your body chemistry. It functions to decrease inflammation and to aid the immune system. However, under situations of constant stress, cortisol be - comes an enemy to health. Excess cortisol over sustained periods of time can increase blood pressure, leading to hypertension, and can cause an imbalance in blood sugar, leading to insulin resistance, diabetes, sleep disturbances, and other problems.

Although normal levels of cortisol help the immune system, increased cortisol levels and decreased DHEA levels can lead to suppression of the immune system (leaving us open to infection and infectious diseases), as well as bone loss, muscular weakening, hardening of the arteries, depression, and increased insulin levels that cause extra fat deposition in the body, especially around the abdomen.[6] Eventually this can lead to heart disease. Stress has been traced as the culprit in flare-ups of arthritis and asthma. Your urinary tract can also be affected. There is a natural balance of friendly and unfriendly organisms that normally coexist in our digestive and urinary systems. Constant anxiety can destroy this balance, however, leading to an overgrowth of the harmful bacteria and yeast.

Even the brain can be affected. Studies have reported that a life of chronic stress may accelerate changes in the brain that lead to memory loss.[7] Stress has a major impact upon nervous system diseases and mental disorders. In particular, the significance of stress in Alzheimer's disease, multiple sclerosis, anxiety, depression, schizophrenia, and post-traumatic stress disorder has been studied.[8]

How Cortisol Works

The adrenal glands help in the regulation of blood pressure and blood mineral content through the secretion of various hormones. They also regulate the body's response to danger or stress. Located above the kidney, their role is to temporarily shift all processes in the body from "maintenance mode" to "high alert." The ensuing rapid heart rate, dry mouth, enhanced mental alertness, and redirection of blood to vital organs are all designed to increase the chances of survival. Today, few of us are chased by saber-toothed tigers or cave bears, but we actually experience much more frequent stressful situations than did early humans. Modern lifestyles produce chronic stress, which creates a constant stimulation of the adrenal glands.

The adrenal glands secrete several hormones. One of these hormones, cortisol, is released as a reaction to stress and in conjunction with sleep-wake patterns. One of the functions of cortisol is to elevate blood sugar (glucose) by breaking down proteins already in the body, such as muscle tissue, as well as fats. These can then be con-

SYMPTOMS OF CORTISOL OVERPRODUCTION

- Depressed immune system
- Increased cholesterol and triglycerides, which increases cardiovascular problems
- Increased blood pressure
- A loss of sex drive
- Sleep disturbances, marked by an inability to "turn off" the day and fall asleep
- Increased weight gain; a breakdown of lean muscle tissue and increase of abdominal fat

- Increased tension, complacency, depression, and irritability
- Down regulation of the thyroid gland, leading to many problems, including an increase in PMS
- Destruction of nerve and brain tissue
- Increased blood sugar (leading to hyper-insulinemia)
- Quickened aging, including premature wrinkling

verted by the liver into glucose. Cortisol also decreases insulin sensitivity of receptor cells, reducing their ability to absorb glucose from the blood and thus increasing blood sugar. Glucose is what the body burns for energy, so this excess glucose can be used for the quick bursts of energy needed to deal with a physical threat. However, few of our modern sources of stress require physical exertion, so we are then left with extra glucose circulating in our veins. And what happens to this extra sugar? That's right; it gets converted into fat and stored. Thus, numerous studies have linked oversecretion of cortisol with obesity and increased fat storage in the body.[9] Eventually, chronic insulin resistance of the receptor cells may turn into type 2 diabetes. With some 16 million diabetics and another 21 million people in the United States with blood sugar and insulin impairment due to various health conditions, this country is on the verge of a medical crisis.[10] One way to help in the prevention of this deadly combination of high insulin levels and poor uptake of glucose is the control of chronic stress through dietary supplementation, exercise, and proper diet.

Cortisol also competes with thyroid hormone for the amino acid tyrosine, which is involved in thyroid hormone formation. Excessive cortisol production therefore limits the amount of thyroid hormone that can be produced. Diminished thyroid hormone may decrease energy and increase fat deposition.

Another unwelcome effect of overactive adrenals due to stress is that it can lead to insomnia. Researchers have found that people with chronic insomnia have increased blood levels of cortisol and another stress hormone called ACTH. Both of these hormones were higher in insomniacs than in control groups. And, in fact, those with the highest levels of cortisol and ACTH had the highest degree of sleep disturbance. Research is also revealing that these hormones are part of the problem with people who have night eating syndrome, which causes an increased appetite at night, especially for carbohydrate-rich foods.[11]

The DHEA Connection

Another hormone produced by the adrenal glands is the steroidal sex hormone DHEA (dehydroepiandrosterone).[12] DHEA is the most abundant steroid in humans, and is synthesized and released primarily by the adrenals, and in small amounts by the brain and skin. It is a precursor for the production of sex hormones, most notably estrogen and testosterone. While the primary role of DHEA is to maintain normal sex hormone levels, it is also thought to combat the effects of stress by balancing cortisol and protecting the immune system. Low levels of DHEA play a role in skin wrinkling, memory decline, and other aging processes.[13] Greater incidence of various cancers, atherosclerosis (hardening of the arteries), and osteoporosis are also associated with a decline in DHEA levels.[14] DHEA increases insulin sensitivity, enhances fat metabolism, and increases antioxidant enzyme synthesis in the liver to protect our bodies against free radical damage.[15] Animal studies suggest that elevating DHEA levels may inhibit breast, colon, and liver cancers, as well as skin tumors.[16] Simply put, healthy DHEA levels help our body combat dreaded enemies of health such as cancer and premature aging.

DHEA is the counterpoint to cortisol: as cortisol levels increase, DHEA levels decline.[17] The primary source of DHEA is pregnen-olone, which is also the precursor for cortisol. During stress or illness, pregnenolone shifts from synthesizing both DHEA and the glucocor-ticoids to producing mainly corticosteroids, such as cortisol. This upsets the ratio of DHEA and cortisol. DHEA levels also are influ-enced by smoking, alcohol consumption, obesity, and chronic illness.

There is now clinical evidence supporting DHEA's use as an anti-aging hormone.[18] In one double-blind, crossover study of 30 sub-jects, age 40 to 70, who received supplements of 50 mg/day DHEA or a placebo for three months, 67 percent of the men and 84 percent of the women in the DHEA group reported a remarkable increase in physical and psychological well-being; no side effects were re-ported.[19] Supporting these results, mice treated with DHEA had glossier coats and less gray hair than control animals.[20] There are reports that treating elderly patients with DHEA supplements often results in improved mood, energy levels, memory, appetite, and skin condition. DHEA has also been reported to increase the body's ability to transform food into energy and burn off excess fat.[21] Another recent finding involves the anti-inflammatory properties of DHEA. It has been known that DHEA can lower the levels of interleukin-6 and tumor necrosis factor alpha, both markers in chronic inflammation. Chronic inflammation is known to play a critical role in the develop-ment of the killer diseases of aging, such as heart disease, Alzheimer's disease, and certain types of cancer.

DHEA supplements are available on the market, but some risks are associated with them. So Relora enters the picture. As we will dis-cuss in more detail in the next chapter, Relora has been reported to increase salivary DHEA levels by 227 percent in patients exposed to mild to moderate stress![22] Maintaining healthy levels of DHEA by using Relora to reduce stress and cortisol levels seems to be the healthiest approach.

Stress and Aging

DHEA is, of course, far from the only factor that affects aging. Researchers increasingly believe that aging begins in our cells, and much of it is due to stress. Let's look at a few facts. The body reaches peak efficiency around age 30 and then declines in many ways. Using age 30 as reflective of 100 percent performance, we see the following: (a) pumping efficiency of the heart is reduced about 20 percent when a person reaches age 55, (b) kidney function is reduced about 25 percent at 55 years of age, (c) maximum breathing capacity declines about 40 percent by age 55 and 60 percent by age 75, and (d) metabolism rate steadily decreases with age.

It is mainly beyond the age of 75 that frailty and the dependence on the medical system associated with chronic illness become apparent. However, with the primary medical problems of the elderly—including diabetes, heart disease, mental confusion, respiratory problems, sexual dysfunction, and cancer—changes in normal body function that contribute to these conditions were going on for many years, below levels of detection. The sooner we identify signs of these disorders, the more likely treatment will be effective. Scientists believe that if we were to arrest these disease processes in our early years, the average life span would be significantly expanded, possibly to as much as 140 years of age! If you can reduce the stress on your cells, then these diseases never get the opportunity to get a foothold, and you prolong your life.

Stress and Gender

While it is true that men may face more immediate life-threatening occupational hazards, women appear to be more vulnerable to stress-induced illnesses, for a variety of reasons. First, they are natural caretakers, and as such they almost automatically take on responsibilities that men might not even consider. This alone adds to the stress loads they carry. Second, men who are stretched thin at their workplaces often go home to relax. Women, on the other hand, go home and keep on working. In spite of the increasing number of women with careers and jobs, traditional roles in their homes still take precedence for many women. They can expect to be in charge of everything from childcare to laundry, food preparation, and social calendars. Given this situation, their minds, as well as their bodies, work overtime. When they become angry about too much to do in too little time with too little help, the anger only adds to their overstressed physical condition. Even women who sense their own need to slow down are programmed toward overcommitment because they feel guilty about not being able to be everything to everyone in their lives. Time spent alone nurturing their own mental and physical well-being might be construed as selfish, so they push even harder on all fronts. Sociologists speculate that many women today may be disadvantaged because they have combined a male standard for achievement in the work world with an old-fashioned female standard for perfection at home.

In women, reduced levels of DHEA caused by stress inhibit their ability to produce the sex hormones estrogen and progesterone, resulting in menstrual abnormalities, premenstrual syndrome, decreased libido, and aggravated menopausal symptoms.[23] A decline in estrogen decreases muscle tone, increases the risk of cardiovascular disease, decreases bone density, and decreases skin tone.[24] Postmeno - pausal decline in estrogen has been associated with an increased risk of Alzheimer's disease.[25] A decline in progesterone can lead to irritability, tension, bloating, headache, loss of sex drive, and increased bone loss.[26] Progesterone also stimulates the shedding of the uterine lining, which prevents uterine hyperplasia, a precancerous condition. Under certain conditions, lack of progesterone increases the risk of uterine cancer.

Men have their own problems associated with low levels of DHEA and the resulting failure to synthesize adequate testosterone. Diminished sex drive, loss of sexual function, decreased muscle mass, depression, cardiovascular disease, and bone loss can all result.[27] It has been demonstrated that men in their forties and fifties can achieve the benefits of testosterone supplementation simply by normalizing their DHEA levels.[28] This may well be accomplished through Relora supplementation.

2. Relora to the Rescue

R elora was developed by Next Pharmaceuticals, a cutting-edge company in Irvine, California dedicated to developing all-natural products for people to achieve optimum health without having to resort to dangerous drugs. The review process they followed to develop Relora included the following elements:

1. A worldwide literature search. This complicated, extensive process, conducted in the English language and by experts trained in Chinese and Japanese, evaluated the world data on stress-relievers in terms of standard results, methods of preparation, chemical compounds in each botanical, structure-activity relationship, and reported pharmacological activity. It focused on plants with known activity that are not widely used in the United States for stress-relief.

2. An assessment of commercial viability, including estimates of availability of ingredients, costs, growing requirements, extraction requirements, and other factors.

Because of their in-depth knowledge of phytochemistry (the chemistry of plants), pharmacology (the effects of drugs on the body), bioavailability (how much is available to be used by the body), toxicology (the toxicity of the agent to the body), and chemistry, the scientists at Next Pharmaceuticals have been able to take this vast amount of knowledge and hone in on a manageable number of plants that can be developed into a safe and effective natural remedy.

Results from Human Trials with Relora

In the first human trial, Relora was tested and found to be a safe, effective, rapid-acting, nonsedating dietary supplement that helps control occasional mild anxiety. Fifty subjects were treated with Relora for two weeks.[29] The dosage was 200 mg of Relora three times daily (the new and improved Relora dosage is 250 mg three times daily). Based on preclinical studies, Relora was designed and evaluated against the following concept—"Relora helps control occasional mild anxiety or mild depression and the associated symptoms: irritability, emotional ups and downs, restlessness, tense muscles, poor sleep, and concentration difficulties." Post-trial analysis revealed an excellent agreement (82 percent) with the pretrial concept. Relaxation was reported by 78 percent of the patients. Relora did not cause significant sedation and 74 percent of the patients had a restful sleep. No significant side effects were reported. Only 24 percent of subjects reported any drowsiness. Relora was gentle on the stomach in 94 percent of the subjects, with only mild and transient gastrointestinal problems in the other 6 percent.

A second trial was undertaken at the Living Longer Wellness Center in Cincinnati, Ohio, to measure cortisol and DHEA levels in 12 patients with mild to moderate stress.[30] A two-week regimen of Relora caused a significant increase in salivary DHEA (227 percent) and a significant decrease in morning salivary cortisol levels (37 percent). Both cortisol and DHEA returned to normal levels in all subjects. These significant findings support Relora's ability to relieve stress and its potential role in weight control and stress-related eating and drinking behavior.

A third human trial with 49 subjects achieved similar results to the first human trial in regards to relaxation and quality of sleep. In addition, Relora was shown to cut stress-related cravings of sweets such as ice cream, cake, pie, and cookies by 76 percent!

A clinical trial on the final formulation of Relora is expected to be completed in 2003.

Can Relora Help Me Lose Weight?

As we've discussed, recent work from the National Institutes of Health (NIH) and other major research centers has demonstrated that stress is a significant contributor to excess body fat.[31] For most people, the primary course of action for losing fat has been exercise and diet alone; for people with elevated cortisol levels, exercise and diet alone may not be enough to achieve their weight-loss goals. By helping the body normalize cortisol and DHEA levels in stressed individuals, Relora may help control weight and stress-related eating or drinking.[32]

A recent study on the stress-induced cortisol cycle confirmed that high-cortisol reactivity in response to stress led to increased eating of high-calorie foods and sweets.[33] Chronic stress can cause cravings for cookies, candy, chips, and other high-fat, high-carbohydrate foods. The stress-driven appetite for these foods leads to dangerous weight gain, primarily around the waist. Sixty percent of American adults are overweight or obese. Stress-related food cravings are certainly one of the factors contributing to this problem. Over 20 percent of American adults are obese with a stress-related condition known as "metabolic syndrome." This condition is characterized by belly fat, high blood pressure, poor cholesterol readings, and high blood sugar. It has been observed in clinical practice that most people feel a major difference within just four weeks of taking Relora, when combined with some simple steps: (a) reduce intake of dairy, wheat, and refined carbohydrates and sugars; (b) decrease red meat consumption; and (c) participate in regular exercise.

Suggested Use and Safety

Safety is of supreme concern when taking any medication or dietary supplement. Even if the agent is effective, if it is not safe, then we must choose another option. The research and development process for Relora was founded on a focus of safety, as well as efficacy, of this unique product. An extensive and elaborate documentation procedure is employed to ensure that each batch of Relora manufactured will be consistent and completely safe when used as directed.

As a dietary supplement, the recommended dosage is 750 mg daily in divided doses: 250 mg three times daily, or 375 mg each morning and evening. Relora can be taken on an empty stomach with water or your favorite beverage, or it can be taken after meals.

Relora is not recommended for use by persons under the age of eighteen. If you are pregnant or nursing, do not take Relora. If you are taking a prescription drug, consult your physician prior to use. Excessive consumption of Relora may impair ability to drive or operate heavy equipment, and it is not recommended for consumption with alcoholic beverages.

3. Complementary Supplements for Stress Relief

While Relora is an exciting breakthrough that can bring improved quality of life to millions of people, it is even more effective at reducing stress levels when combined with additional supplementation and simple lifestyle changes. This chapter explains the vitamins, minerals, herbs, and practices you might want to consider using with Relora if stress is an issue in your life.

B Vitamins

The vitamin B complex, consisting of eleven separate vitamins, plays an important role in the support of a healthy nervous system. All of the B vitamins are known to aid the functions of the brain and nervous system. The B vitamins are also known as the "antistress" vitamins. One of the most important may be B_5, or pantothenic acid. Vitamin B_5 depletion is associated with stress, nervous irritability, and adrenal exhaustion. Vitamin B_5 is involved in the production of adrenal hormones, and B_5 deficiency causes a progressive decline in the production of adrenal hormones.[34]

Vitamin B_6 (pyridoxine) may affect mood through its important role in processing beneficial series-one prostaglandins.[35] Vitamin B_6 is used for depression in menopausal women,[36] and is associated with the synthesis of serotonin, dopamine, and gamma-amino butyric acid (GABA).[37] A deficiency of vitamin B_6 has been shown to cause muscle weakness, fatigue, irritability, and depression.[38] Some medications may cause a depletion of this vitamin, including antibiotics[39] and estrogen-containing medications including oral contraceptives and estrogen replacement therapy.[40] Check with your doctor or pharmacist if medications you are taking may deplete this vitamin. Vitamin B_{12} is essential in the metabolism of the nerve tissue and necessary for the health of the entire nervous system, as it nourishes the myelin sheaths that insulate conduction in the nerves.[41] Slightly low levels of niacin (B_3) may lead to depression, apprehension, hyperirritability, emotional instability, and impairment of recent memory.[42] Thiamine (B_1) deficiency has been shown to cause lethargy and fatigue.[43] As shown in one study, subjects with low folate (another B vitamin) levels were more likely to have melancholic depression and were significantly less likely to respond to Prozac.[44] Findings link low folate levels to poorer response to antidepressant treatment, and folate levels might be considered in the evaluation of depressed patients who do not respond to antidepressant treatment. Medications may also deplete the body of this vitamin, including oral contraceptives and antibiotics.[45] Due to the many factors that may be affecting our B vitamin intake (stress, prescription drugs, inadequate dietary intake), a multivitamin or a B-complex supplement may be needed to ensure adequate intake. (Caution: side effects may occur with doses greater than recommended of vitamin B_3 and B_6.) If you're taking a multivitamin already, check the doses of the B vitamins and adjust accordingly. The total daily dosages you should be taking are:

- Vitamin B_1 (thiamine):   5–10 mg

- Vitamin B_2 (riboflavin):   5–10 mg

- Vitamin B_3 (niacin):   25–100 mg

- Vitamin B_5 (pantothenic acid):   10–50 mg

- Vitamin B_6 (pyridoxine):   10–20 mg

- Vitamin B_{12} (cyanocobalamin):   500 mcg

Vitamin C

Vitamin C is an important antistress antioxidant. The adrenal glands are dependent upon certain vital nutrients to maintain healthy output of adrenal hormones and adequate response to stress. Vitamin C is one of those nutrients because it directly supports the production of stress hormones, and can become depleted during times of stress, thereby lowering the body's supply of this nutrient, which is also important for resistance to infection and for protecting cells from free-radical damage. Recent research shows that large doses of vitamin C reduce the levels of stress hormones in the bloodstream, allowing the body's immune system to work more efficiently and helping to prevent diseases ranging from colds to cancer. Scientists subjected laboratory rats to stress and then gave the animals huge doses of vitamin C—the equivalent of a human eating several thousand milligrams of the vitamin.[46] The vitamin C significantly reduced the levels of stress hormones in the rats' blood. The vitamin C treatment also reduced the other typical indicators of physical and emotional stress, including weight loss, enlarged adrenal glands, and changes in the thymus and spleen, which help produce immune cells. The most common dosage of vitamin C is 250 mg daily, but doses up to 2 grams may be necessary. As with other nutrients, some medications may cause a depletion of this vitamin, including aspirin and oral contraceptives.[47]

Minerals

Calcium and magnesium are important antistress minerals. Magnesium slows the release of the neurochemicals epinephrine and norepinephrine from the adrenal glands, which makes it a critical mineral for balancing the sympathetic nervous system ("fight or flight") response.[48] Magnesium also helps decrease insulin resistance and stabilizes blood sugar, which is important in counteracting the effects of cortisol.[49] Magnesium increases HDL cholesterol (the "good" cholesterol) concentration in the blood and balances the cellular absorption of calcium. Symptoms of magnesium deficiency include anxiety, restlessness, nervousness, fatigue, leg cramps, muscle weakness, heart palpitations, and insomnia. Severe magnesium loss can result in irregular heart rhythms. Statistics show that 75 percent of Americans are low in magnesium or are getting below the Recommended Dietary Allowance.[50] Many people suffering from anxiety, nervousness, and sleep problems may find real help by taking magnesium. Look for the citrate, aspartate, or glycinate forms of magnesium.

Calcium is the most abundant mineral in the human body. Average healthy males have two-and-a-half to three pounds of calcium while females have about two pounds. Approximately 99 percent of our calcium is located in the bones and teeth, which leaves only a trace in our cells and body fluids. While the most important function of calcium involves the maintenance of skeletal health, the small percentage of calcium outside the bones is used to maintain a variety of vital body functions.[51] Calcium is necessary to initiate muscle contractions, thereby playing a vital role in maintaining a healthy heartbeat.[52] Calcium helps maintain proper transmission of nerve impulses, thereby being important in stressful situations.[53] On the cellular level, calcium is a major factor in the regulation of the passage of nutrients and wastes through cell membranes. It is also involved in the regulation of various enzymes that control muscle contraction, fat digestion, and metabolism.

Zinc, selenium, copper, and manganese are minerals important for the support of enzymes. Zinc alone is involved in hundreds of enzymatic reactions, including those involved in adrenal activity.[54] Zinc is extremely important for the immune function, specifically the production of T cells from the thymus. High levels of cortisol deplete zinc stores.[55] Elevated cortisol and ACTH have been linked to thymus atrophy and shrinkage, and depression of T-cell production. Corticosteroid therapy increases the need for a host of other nutrients, including calcium, folic acid, magnesium, potassium, selenium, vitamins C and D, and zinc.

Antioxidant Nutrients

It is well documented that oxidative stress is a cellular or physiological condition that results in damage to vital structures and functions in the body.[56] A wide range of factors such as air pollution, alcohol, cigarette smoke, nonionizing radiation, and psychological stress seem to increase oxidative stress. To reduce cellular damages associated with oxidative stress, it is important to ingest adequate levels of antioxidant nutrients from a combination of dietary sources and nutritional supplements. Some of the most important antioxidants for consideration include the aforementioned vitamin C, vitamin E, vitamin A (beta-carotene), selenium, coenzyme Q_{10}, alpha lipoic acid, acetyl 1-carnitine, and the herbs bilberry, grapeseed extract, green tea, and milk thistle, to name a few. The level of antioxidant nutrients for supplementation will vary greatly depending on the cumulative overall levels of stress and the biochemical makeup of the individual. However, due to the many factors that can lead to oxidative stress in the body, finding a well-rounded antioxidant supplement is needed to help neutralize their effects.

Panax Ginseng (*Panax quinquifolium*)

The ginsengs are some of the most frequently purchased herbal supplements in the United States. Historically, panax ginseng, or Asian ginseng, has been used for a variety of health benefits, especially for its adaptogenic and tonic effects for people fatigued or under stress.[57] Panax ginseng is an adaptogen. It has a nonspecific action on the body that increases its ability to cope with various stressors, including physiological, emotional, and external toxins, thus reducing susceptibility to illness.

It is thought that ginsenosides (the active constituents in panax ginseng) act at hormone receptor sites, especially in the hypothalamus and pituitary glands, stimulating secretion of ACTH.[58] ACTH stimulates the production of adrenal hormones and other factors, leading to balance and regulation of the hypothalamic/adrenal axis that may have been influenced by stress. The dosage of panax ginseng for use in stress is 200–600 mg daily, standardized to contain a minimum of 5 percent ginsenosides. If panax ginseng is used as stress support, a regimen of three weeks on, two weeks off is best. It may take several weeks for a clinical effect to become apparent.

Ashwagandha (*Withania somnifera*)

Ashwagandha root, also known as winter cherry or Indian ginseng, is an important herb from India's Ayurvedic system of medicine. Ashwagandha has been traditionally used for the treatment of debility, emaciation, impotence, and premature aging.[59] This dietary supplement is used to enhance mental and physical performance, improve learning ability, and decrease stress and fatigue. Ashwagandha is a general tonic to be used in stressful situations, especially insomnia, overwork, nervousness, and restlessness. The recommended dosage of ashwagandha is 450 mg two or three times daily, standardized to contain 1.5 percent withanolides per dose.

Rhodiola (*Rhodiola rosea*)

Rhodiola, or Arctic root, has been used in traditional folk medicine in China, Serbia, and the Carpathian Mountains of the Ukraine. In the former Soviet Union, it has been used as an adaptogen, decreasing fatigue and increasing the body's natural resistance to various stresses. In Siberia, it is said that those who drink rhodiola tea regularly will live more than a hundred years. Rhodiola seems to enhance the body's physical and mental work capacity and productivity, with actions related to strengthening the nervous system, fighting depression, enhancing immunity, elevating the capacity for exercise, enhancing memorization, improving energy levels, and possibly prolonging lifespan.[60] In Mongolia, it was used for the treatment of tuberculosis and cancer. In animal experiments, rhodiola extract increased blood insulin and decreased glucagon levels, resulting in a 50 to 80 percent increase in liver glycogen. This information suggests that rhodiola extracts may help normalize blood sugar levels and decrease insulin resistance.[61] The recommended dosage of rhodiola is 50–100 mg twice a day, standardized to contain 1 percent salidrosid or 40–50 percent phenylpropenoids per dose.

Relaxation

Stress often manifests itself as muscle tension and tightness. This is a manifestation of the sympathetic nervous system, which dominates during times of stress. Even if stress is unavoidable, it is possible to reduce the tension associated with it by engaging the parasympathetic nervous system. When relaxed, the parasympathetic nervous system, which is designed to promote repair, maintenance, and restoration, is in charge. Relaxation exercises, meditation, yoga, tai chi, and massage can all promote the parasympathetic response and assist in relieving the physical signs of stress.

There are infinite ways to begin to relax, you just have to make the effort. Gardening calms people, as do pets. It is impossible to be relaxed and stressed at the same time. By guiding oneself into relaxation, stress is forced to subside. There is no way to do justice to stress-relieving techniques in this booklet—it would take many more chapters. Search the Internet, look in your library, check out bulletin boards—you will find multiple options for stress management.

The following relaxation technique can be used any time. Find a quiet place to sit. Begin by taking a few deep, slow breaths. Beginning with the hands and arms, contract the muscles to about three-quarters of their maximum tension, then relax. Continue progressing to the feet, legs, torso, and face. Inhale and exhale slowly during this exercise. The exercise can be completed in less than fifteen minutes and the effect is remarkable. Structure your time to complete a relaxation exercise a few times a day if possible. If this does not realistically fit your lifestyle, make sure that you have time to do activities that serve no other purpose than to provide joy and laughter.

Sleep

Poor sleep habits contribute to stress, irritability, and depression. New evidence actually links sleep deprivation with diabetes, obesity, and other health conditions. Sleep deprivation interferes with productivity, which can further aggravate stress. Inadequate sleep can also interfere with immune function and lead to the physical stress of illness. The most restful sleep is roughly between 9 P.M. and 9 A.M. This means that eight hours of sleep (give or take a couple) between 10 P.M. and 6 A.M. are more restorative than the same sleep from 3 A.M. to 11 A.M. Napping during the day can help make up for sleep deprivation, but may interfere with falling asleep in the evening. Ultimately, you are cheating yourself if you try to beat the sleep clock. Those who fall prey to deadlines and commitments, slipping into bad sleep habits, inevitably pay the price.

Exercise

Exercise is a very effective tool for helping to manage stress because it lowers elevated cortisol. In addition, it decreases insulin resistance and helps end the vicious cycles of stress eating and insulin resistance-induced weight gain. While full-scale discussion of all the physical benefits of exercise is impossible within the scope of this book, we hope to give you enough information to help you realize that consistent exercise will help you get started in regaining control of your metabolism.

Heavy exercise is a form of physical stress that can have a negative impact on your health if you do not take steps to replenish the accelerated nutrient loss, free radical damage, and wear and tear on your frame. Most experts agree that light to moderate exercise can diminish mental and emotional stress and have a positive impact on your metabolism without heightening risk of injury. Moderate exercise reduces the effects of stress hormones by providing a physical outlet for stressful feelings. Aerobic exercise stimulates the release of endorphins from the pituitary and hypothalamus. Endorphins bind with opiate receptors in the brain to relieve pain and promote a sense of well-being. There is some evidence that exercise training increases circulating DHEA, even while you are at rest.[62] Exercise also has a significant impact on blood sugar. By controlling blood sugar more effectively, you are managing a key factor in the development of diabetes and obesity. In addition, proper exercise and stretching keeps you limber as you age, builds bone density, and makes you feel better mentally. Regular exercise has even been reported to help people who are depressed overcome their depression. The physiological changes associated with exercise contribute to an overall sense of control, health, and ability to cope with stress.

Conclusion

Stress—even the word makes us feel anxiety! As we've looked into the causes, symptoms, and long-term effects of this killer, it's become clear how important stress-regulation is, especially as we get older. Thanks to stress, our memory fades, we get aches and pains in places we hadn't noticed before, we don't sleep, and we gain weight. We also begin to see wrinkles in our skin, around the eyes, on our forehead, and around our mouth. Our hair turns prematurely gray. During chronic stress, we may begin to overeat and crave certain foods high in sugar. Some of us even develop type 2 diabetes, high blood pressure, high cholesterol levels, and other serious health problems, including cancer. Control stress, and we push back the age clock.

Because it is a natural, safe, nonsedating, and effective ingredient, Relora offers many advantages to the health consumer seeking a natural way to deal with stress and anxiety, stress-related weight gain, or symptoms of premature aging. The potential health benefits of Relora are not currently available from any other product. Relora can now be found as a stand-alone dietary supplement or as an ingredient in other dietary supplement formulas. Try it and begin your embrace of a long, beautiful, and stress-free life.

Notes

1. Niwa Y, et al. *Protection for Life: How to Boost Your Body's Defenses Against Free Radicals and the Aging Effects of Pollution and Modern Lifestyles.* Wellingborough, UK: Thorsons, (1989), 9.

2. Ritter C, Hobfoll SE, et al. Stress, psychosocial resources, and depressive symptomatology during pregnancy in low-income, inner-city women. *Health Psychol.* 19 (Nov 2000): 576–85.

3. Sufka KJ, Roach JT, Chambliss WG, et al. Anxiolytic properties of botanical extracts in the chick social separation-stress procedure. *Psychopharmacology* 153 (Jan 1, 2001): 219–24.

4. Nick GL. Stress-related eating and metabolic syndrome: an important cause of obesity among women. *Townsend Letter* (Dec 2002): 50–52.

5. Ibid.

6. Epel E, Lapidus R, McEwen B, et al. Stress may add bite to appetite in women: a laboratory study of stress-induced cortisol and eating behavior. *Psychoneuroendocrinology* 26 (Jan 2001): 37–49; Vanitallie TB. Stress: a risk factor for serious illness. *Metabolism* 51 (Jun 2002): 40–45; Paik IH, Toh KY, Lee C, et al. Psychological stress may induce increased humoral and decreased cellular immunity. *Behav Med.* 26 (Fall 2000): 139–41; McEwen BS. The neurobiology of stress: from serendipity to clinical relevance. *Brain Res.* 886 (Dec 15, 2000):172–89.

7. Moulds ML, Bryant RA. Directed forgetting in acute stress disorder. *J Abnorm Psychol.* 111 (Feb 2002): 175–79; Kim JJ, Diamond DM. The stressed hippocampus, synaptic plasticity and lost memories. *Nat Rev Neurosci.* 3 (Jun 2002): 453–62.

8. Esch T, Stefano GB, Fricchione GL, et al. The role of stress in neurodegenerative diseases and mental disorders. *Neuroendocrinol Lett.* 23 (Jun 2002): 199–208.

9. Maarin P, Darin N, Amemiya T, Andersson B, Jern S, Bjaorntorp P. Cortisol secretion in relation to body fat distribution in obese premenopausal women. *Metabolism* 41 (1992): 882–86.

10. Harris MI, et al. Early detection of undiagnosed diabetes mellitus: a U.S. perspective. *Diabetes Metab Res Rev* 16 (Jul/Aug 2000): 230–36.

11. Birketvedt GS, Sunsfjord J, Florholmen JR. Hypothalmic-pituitary-adrenal axis in the night eating syndrome. *Am J Physiol Endocrinol Metab* 2002 Feb;282(2):e366–9; *Journal of Clinical Endocrinology and Metabolism* 2001 August;86:3787–3794.

12. Bradlow HL, Murphy J, Byrne JJ. Immunological properties of dehydroepiandrosterone, its conjugates, and metabolites. *Ann NY Acad Sci* 876 (Jun 22, 1999): 91–101.

13. Lee KS, Oh KY, Kim BC. Effects of dehydroepiandrosterone on collagen and collagenase gene expression by skin fibroblasts in culture. *J Dermatol Sci.* 23 (Jun 2000):103–10; Phillips TJ, Demircay Z, Sahu M. Hormonal effects on skin aging. *Clin Geriatr Med.* 17 (Nov 2001): 661–72.

14. Urban RJ. Neuroendocrinology of aging in the male and female. *Endocrinol Metab Clin North Am.* 21 (Dec 1992): 921–31; Ledochowski M, Murr C, Jager M, et al. Dehydroepiandrosterone, aging and immune activation. *Exp Gerontol.* 36 (Nov 2001): 1739–47.

15. Schauer JE, Schelin A, Hanson P, et al. Dehydroepiandrosterone and a beta-agonist, energy transducers, alter antioxidant enzyme systems: influence of chronic training and acute exercise in rats. *Arch Biochem Biophys* 283 (Dec 1990): 503–11; Buffington CK, Pourmotabbed G, Kitabchi AE. Case report: amelioration of insulin resistance in diabetes with dehydroepiandrosterone. *Am J Med Sci* 306 (Nov 1993): 320–24; Casson PR, et al. Replacement of dehydroepiandrosterone enhances T-lymphocyte insulin binding in postmenopausal women. *Fertil Steril* 63 (May 1995): 1027–31; Mukasa K, et al. Dehydroepiandrosterone (DHEA) ameliorates the insulin sensitivity in older rats. *J Steroid Biochem Mol Biol* 67 (Nov 1998): 355–58; De Pergola G. The adipose tissue metabolism: role of testosterone and dehydroepiandrosterone. *Int J Obes Relat Metab Disord* 24 (S2) (Jun 2000): 59–63S; Khalil A, et al. Age-related decrease of dehydroepiandrosterone concentrations in low density lipoproteins and its role in the susceptibility of low density lipoproteins to lipid peroxidation. *J Lipid Res* 4 (Oct 2000): 1552–61.

16. Nyce JW, Magee DN, Hard GC, Schwartz AG. Inhibition on 1,2-dimethylhydrazine-induced colon tumorigenesis in Balb/c mice by dehy-

droepiandrosterone. *Carcinogenesis* 5 (1984): 57–62; Mayer D, et al. Modulation of liver carcinogenesis by dehydroepiandrosterone. In: Kalimi M, Regelson W, eds. *The Biologic Role of Dehydroepiandrosterone (DHEA)*. New York: Walter de Gruyter, 1990, 361–85; Schwartz AG. Inhibition of spontaneous breast cancer formation in female C3H (Avy/a) mice by long-term treatment with dehydroepiandrosterone. *Cancer Res* 39 (1979): 1129–32.

17. Yamakita N, Murai T, Kokubo Y, et al. Dehydroepiandrosterone sulphate is increased and dehydroepiandrosterone response to corticotrophin-releasing hormone is decreased in the hyperthyroid state compared with the euthyroid state. *Clin Endocrinol* 55 (Dec 2001): 797–803.

18. Johnson MD, Bebb RA, Sirrs SM. Uses of DHEA in aging and other disease states. *Aging Res Rev.* 1 (Feb 2002): 29–41.

19. Yen SS, Morales AJ, Khorrram O. Replacement of DHEA in aging men and women. Potential remedial effects. *Ann NY Acad Sci* 774 (1995): 128–42.

20. Bosse K, Fehr R, Franz E, et al. [Effects of dehydroepiandrosterone-sulfate on hair growth in mice and guinea pigs]. *Arch Dermatol Forsch.* 243 (1972): 177–87.

21. Abate N, Haffner SM, Garg A, et al. Sex steroid hormones, upper body obesity, and insulin resistance. *J Clin Endocrinol Metab.* 87 (Oct 2002): 4522–27.

22. Nick GL. Stress-related eating and metabolic syndrome: an important cause of obesity among women. *Townsend Letter* (Dec 2002): 50–52.

23. Burger HG, Dudley EC, Robertson DM, et al. Hormonal changes in the menopause transition. *Recent Prog Horm Res.* 57 (2002): 257–75.

24. Harlow BL, Signorello LB. Factors associated with early menopause. *Maturitas.* 42 (S1) (Jun 15, 2002): S87–93.

25. Ibid.

26. Burger HG, Dudley EC, Robertson DM, et al. Hormonal changes in the menopause transition. *Recent Prog Horm Res.* 57 (2002): 257–75.

27. Van den Beld AW, Lamberts SW. Endocrine aspects of healthy ageing in men. *Novartis Found Symp.* 242 (2002): 3–25.

28. Morales AJ, Nolan JJ, Nelson LC, et al. Effects of replacement dose of dehydroepiandrosterone in men and women of advancing age. *J Clin Endo - crinol Metab* 78 (Jun 1994): 1360–67.

29. Nick GL. Stress-related eating and metabolic syndrome: an important cause of obesity among women. *Townsend Letter* (Dec 2002): 50–52.

30. Ibid.

31. Cohen M, Klein E, Kuten A, et al. Increased emotional distress in daughters of breast cancer patients is associated with decreased natural cytotoxic activity, elevated levels of stress hormones and decreased secretion of Th1 cytokines. *Int J Cancer* 100 (Jul 20, 2002): 347–54; Pasquali R, Anconetani B, Chattat R, et al. Hypothalamic-pituitary-adrenal axis activity and its relationship to the autonomic nervous system in women with visceral and subcutaneous obesity: effects of the corticotropin-releasing factor/argininevasopressin test and of stress. *Metabolism* 45 (Mar 1996): 351–56; Tremblay A, Doucet E. Obesity: a disease or a biological adaptation? *Obes Rev.* 1 (May 2000): 27–35.

32. Homma M, Oka K, Niitsuma T, et al. A novel 11 beta-hydroxysteroid dehydrogenase inhibitor contained in saiboku-to, a herbal remedy for steroid-dependent bronchial asthma. *J Pharm Pharmacol.* 46 (Apr 1994): 305–09.

33. Epel E, Lapidus R, McEwen B, Brownell K. Stress may add bite to appetite in women: a laboratory study of stress-induced cortisol and eating behavior. *Psychoneuroendocrinology* 26 (Jan 2001): 37–49.

34. Lesser M. *Nutrition and Vitamin Therapy.* New York: Grove Press, 1980, 69–70.

35. Henrotte JG, et al. Effect of pyridoxine on mice gastric ulcers and brain catecholamines after an immobilization stress. *Ann Nutr Metab.* 36 (1992): 313–17; Lindenbaum ES, et al. Effects of pyridoxine on mice after immobilization stress. *Nutr Metab.* 17 (1974): 368–74.

36. Brush MG, et al. Pyridoxine in the treatment of premenstrual syndrome: a retrospective survey in 630 patients. *Br J Clin Pract* 42 (1988): 448–52.

37. Dolphin, et al (eds). *Vitamin B$_6$: Pyridoxal Phosphate.* Toronto, ON: John Wiley and Sons, 1986.

38. Merrill AH, et al. Diseases associated with defects in vitamin B$_6$ metabolism or utilization. *Annu Rev Nutr.* 7 (1987): 137–56.

39. Cummings JH, Macfarlane G. Role of intestinal bacteria in nutrient metabolism. *J Parenter Enteral Nutr.* 21 (1997): 357–65.

40. Haspels AA, et al. Disturbance of tryptophan metabolism and its correction during oestrogen treatment in postmenopausal women. *Maturitas* 1 (1978): 15–20.

41. Bottiglieri T. Folate, Vitamin B$_{12}$, and Neuropsychiatric Disorders. *Nutr Rev* 54 (1996): 382–90.

42. Machlin LJ. New views on the function and health effects of vitamins. *Nutrition* 10 (1994): 562.

43. Anderson GH. Diet, neurotransmitters and brain function. *Br Med Bull.* 37 (1981): 95–100.

44. Fava M, et al. Folate, vitamin B$_{12}$, and homocysteine in major depressive disorder. *Am J Psychiatry* 154 (1977): 426–28.

45. Webb JL. Nutritional effects of oral contraceptive use: a review. *J Reprod Med.* 25 (Oct 1980): 150–56; Cummings JH, Macfarlane G. Role of intestinal bacteria in nutrient metabolism. *J Parenter Enteral Nutr.* 21 (1977): 357–65.

46. Kojo S, Tanaka K, et al. [Oxidative stress and vitamins]. *Nippon Rinsho.* 57 (Oct 1999): 2325–31.

47. Sahud MA, et al. Effect of aspirin ingestion on ascorbic-acid levels in rheumatoid arthritis. *Lancet* 7706 (1971): 937–38; Webb JL. Nutritional effects of oral contraceptive use: a review. *J Reprod Med.* 25 (1980): 150–56.

48. Chakraborti S, Chakraborti T, Mandal M, et al. Protective role of magnesium in cardiovascular diseases: a review. *Mol Cell Biochem.* 238 (Sep 2002): 163–79.

49. Golf SW, Bender S, Gruttner J. On the significance of magnesium in extreme physical stress. *Cardiovasc Drugs Ther.* 12 (S2) (Sep 1998): 197–202.

50. Cohen L. The role of magnesium. *Isr Med Assoc J.* 4 (Mar 2002): 232–33.

51. Anderson JJ. Calcium requirements during adolescence to maximize bone health. *J Am Coll Nutr.* 20 (S2) (Apr 2001): 186S–191S.

52. McCarron DA, et al. Are low intakes of calcium and potassium important causes of cardiovascular disease? *Am J Hypertens.* 14 (S2) (Jun 2001): 206S–212S.

53. Augustine GJ. How does calcium trigger neurotransmitter release? *Curr Opin Neurobiol.* 11 (Jun 2001): 320–26.

54. Aggett PJ. Physiology and metabolism of essential trace elements: an outline. *Clin Endocrinol Metab.* 14 (Aug 1985): 513–43.

55. Gleason M, Bishop NC. Elite athlete immunology: importance of nutrition. *Int J Sports Med.* 21 (S1) (May 2000): S44–50.

56. Polidori MC, Mecocci P, et al. Physical activity and oxidative stress during aging. *Int J Sports Med.* 21 (Apr 2000): 154–57.

57. Bradley PR, ed. *British Herbal Compendium, vol. 1.* Bournemouth, UK: British Herbal Medicine Association, 1992, 115–17.

58. Hiai S, et al. Stimulation of pituitary-adrenocortical system by ginseng saponin. *Endocrinol Jpn.* 26 (1979): 661–65.

59. Boone K. Withania—the Indian ginseng and anti-aging adaptogen. *Nutrition and Healing* 5 (Jun 1998): 5–7.

60. Rege NN, et al. Adaptogenic properties of six Rasayana herbs used in Ayurvedic Medicine. *Phytother Res.* 13 (Jun 1999): 275–91.

61. Molokovskii DS, et al. [The action of adaptogenic plant preparations in experimental alloxan diabetes]. *Probl Endokrinol.* 35 (Nov/Dec 1989): 82–87.

62. Flaire E, Duche P, Lac G. Effects of amount of training on the saliva concentrations of cortisol, dehydroepiandrosterone, and on the dehydroepiandrosterone-cortisol concentration ratio in women over 16 weeks of training. *Eur J Appl Physiol Occup Physiol* 78 (Oct 1998): 466–71.

Resources

Relora is now available in most health-food stores and pharmacies. For information on ordering Relora directly from manufacturers, please visit:

www.relora.com

Index

About the Author

James B. LaValle, R.Ph., C.N.C., has been involved with natural medicine for the past fifteen years. Known as *America's Pharmacist,* he is a nationally recognized figure in the field of natural therapeutics. Dr. LaValle is the author of several books, including *Smart Medicine for Healthier Living* and *Drug-Induced Nutrient Depletion Handbook.*

Printed in the USA
CPSIA information can be obtained
at www.ICGtesting.com
JSHW012010140824
68134JS00004B/104

9 781681 627762